KINESIOLOGY TAPING GUIDE FOR WOMEN

Empowering Women Through Kinesiology, A Comprehensive Guide to Optimal Health and Performance

ANDREW KATE

Copyright © 2023

All Rights Are Reserved

The content in this book may not be reproduced, duplicated, or transferred without the express written permission of the author or publisher. Under no circumstances will the publisher or author be held liable or legally responsible for any losses, expenditures, or damages incurred directly or indirectly as a consequence of the information included in this book.

Legal Remarks

Copyright protection applies to this publication. It is only intended for personal use. No piece of this work may be modified, distributed, sold, quoted, or paraphrased without the author's or publisher's consent.

Disclaimer Statement

Please keep in mind that the contents of this booklet are meant for educational and recreational purposes. Every effort has been made to offer accurate, up-to-date, reliable, and thorough information. There are, however, no stated or implied assurances of any kind. Readers understand that the author is providing competent counsel. The content in this book originates from several sources. Please seek the opinion of a competent professional before using any of the tactics outlined in this book. By reading this book, the reader agrees that the author will not be held accountable for any direct or indirect damages resulting from the use of the information contained therein, including, but not limited to, errors, omissions, or inaccuracies.

TABLE OF CONTENTS

INTRODUCTION

While aging offers a multitude of experiences and wisdom, it also presents new obstacles to one's physical health. Seniors' quality of life is frequently impacted by joint stiffness, decreased mobility, and muscular soreness. Kinesiology taping is a potent, non-invasive technique that helps seniors maintain an active and satisfying lifestyle by assisting them on their path to improved mobility and health.

Kinesiology Taping: An Overview

Kinesiology tape is a therapeutic method based on an understanding of human anatomy and movement, not just putting adhesive strips on the skin. The goal of this book is to explore the concepts and methods of kinesiology taping that are especially designed to meet the special requirements of elderly people. Through the application of elasticity, support, and proprioception, kinesiology tape is a multipurpose tool that helps the elderly move more functionally, heal more quickly, and have less discomfort.

Kinesiology Taping's Benefits for Seniors

Seniors have a variety of musculoskeletal problems, such as arthritis, decreased joint stability, poor posture, and decreased mobility. Kinesiology taping provides a mild yet efficient way to deal with these issues. Because of its non-restrictive character and capacity to enhance the effects of other therapies, it is the perfect adjuvant for improving seniors' general well-being. Seniors can participate in everyday activities with more ease and confidence when they use kinesiology tape to support weak muscles, improve circulation, and reduce discomfort.

Using This Navigation Guide

This extensive manual is designed to give seniors and caregivers insightful knowledge about the uses, advantages, and subtleties of kinesiology taping. Each chapter provides a multitude of information and helpful advice, covering anything from the basic ideas underlying taping procedures to particular strategies aimed at typical senior difficulties. A comprehensive grasp of this therapeutic method is also provided by exploring advanced approaches, cautionary concerns, and real-life instances.

Senior Empowerment for Optimal Health

Beyond just applying tape, this guide aims to educate elders by empowering them to take an active role in their own wellness journey by empowering them to understand their bodies. Seniors may benefit from increased mobility, less discomfort, and a fresh sense of independence by incorporating the ideas and techniques presented in this guide, which will allow them to face a life full of energy and vitality.

This introduction lays the groundwork for a thorough investigation of the ways in which kinesiology taping can improve seniors' health and well-being, with a focus on empowerment, comprehension, and real-world application for an improved standard of living.

CHAPTER ONE

INTRODUCTION TO KINESIOLOGY TAPING

Understanding Kinesiology Taping

Using elastic adhesive strips to the skin, kinesiology taping is a therapeutic method that supports muscles and joints without limiting movement. Kinesiology tape functions by interacting with the body's sensory receptors, influencing the neurological system, and fostering a variety of physiological outcomes, in contrast to typical athletic taping, which primarily focuses on stabilization.

Kinesiology Taping's Foundational Ideas

1. Elasticity: Kinesiology tape's special elasticity resembles the suppleness of human skin. This characteristic permits a complete range of motion while maintaining the stability and support of muscles and joints.

2. Support and Stability: Kinesiology tape provides space by gently raising the skin, which can lessen pressure on pain receptors and ease discomfort. It improves function by providing support to weaker joints or muscles without limiting movement.

3. Enhancement of Proprioception: Applying the tape can improve proprioception, or the body's knowledge of its spatial orientation. Increased bodily awareness and improved muscular coordination may result from this increased sensory input.

The Operation of Kinesiology Taping

Kinesiology tape application requires precise techniques that take into account the body's positioning, tension, and direction. When used correctly, the tape can impose different levels of skin stress, which can affect muscle function, circulation, and the feeling of pain. Users may profit from this procedure in a number of ways, including:

Pain Relief: Kinesiology tape can ease the discomfort brought on by a number of conditions by enhancing circulation and releasing pressure from pain receptors.

Muscle Support: By improving muscle function and lowering tiredness, the tape helps people participate in activities with a lower risk of strain or injury.

Improving Circulation and Swelling: Its application methods may help to enhance lymphatic and blood circulation, which may lessen swelling and hasten the healing process after injuries.

Posture and Movement Enhancement: Kinesiology tape can help with posture correction and better movement patterns by influencing proprioception and muscle support.

Velocity and Flexibility

The adaptability of kinesiology taping is a major benefit. It can be customized to treat a range of ailments, from recent wounds to long-term problems, and it can be utilized in addition to other therapeutic approaches.

Thoughts and Safety Measures

Even though kinesiology taping is usually thought to be safe, correct application is essential to enjoying its benefits. Before using it, people with specific skin disorders or allergies should use caution or consult a healthcare provider. To further prevent negative consequences, it is essential to learn proper application procedures and optimum tension levels.

Benefits for Senior Individuals

Seniors can benefit from kinesiology tapping in a number of ways that are specific to their physical needs and age-related difficulties.

1. Pain Alleviation and Management

Relieving Arthritis: Seniors frequently experience pain from arthritis. When used properly, kinesiology tape can reduce pain by improving circulation, lessening pressure on delicate areas, and gently supporting afflicted joints.

Relief from Chronic Pain: By modifying pain signals and providing targeted support to strained or weakening muscles, kinesiology tape can help manage chronic pain resulting from age-related disorders or musculoskeletal problems.

2. Improved Usability and Mobility

Combined Assistance: Kinesiology tape offers additional support that can be beneficial for seniors who are experiencing joint instability or weakness. It can aid in joint stabilization, resulting in increased mobility and a lower chance of damage when moving.

Enhanced Flexibility: Kinesiology tape supports muscles and encourages improved movement patterns, allowing seniors to maintain or improve their range of motion without being restrictive.

3. Support and Posture Correction

Postural Improvement: By providing subtle signals to promote better alignment and lessening pressure on muscles and joints, kinesiology tape application techniques can help correct bad posture that is frequently observed in seniors.

Improving Balance: The proprioceptive effects of the tape can help seniors become more balanced and stable, which may lower their chance of falling, which is a major worry for this population.

4. Supplemental Rehab and Wellbeing Instrument

Aide for Rehabilitation: Kinesiology tape can support specific muscles or joints in seniors receiving physical therapy or rehabilitation, which can improve the efficacy of exercises and therapies.

Inclusive Choice: Kinesiology taping is especially intriguing to seniors who prefer natural approaches to managing their health and fitness because it is a non-invasive and drug-free procedure.

5. Health of the Mind

Increased Confidence: Kinesiology tape can help seniors feel more confident about their capacity to participate in everyday activities by offering support and pain relief. This can promote independence and a positive view of their skills.

Safety Considerations and Precautions

Seniors can benefit from kinesiology tapping in a number of ways that are specific to their physical needs and age-related difficulties.

1. Pain Alleviation and Management

Relieving Arthritis: Seniors frequently experience pain from arthritis. When used properly, kinesiology tape can reduce pain by improving circulation, lessening pressure on delicate areas, and gently supporting afflicted joints.

Relief from Chronic Pain: By modifying pain signals and providing targeted support to strained or weakening muscles, kinesiology tape can help manage chronic pain resulting from age-related disorders or musculoskeletal problems.

2. Improved Usability and Mobility

Combined Assistance: Kinesiology tape offers additional support that can be beneficial for seniors who are experiencing joint instability or weakness. It can aid in joint stabilization, resulting in increased mobility and a lower chance of damage when moving.

Enhanced Flexibility: Kinesiology tape supports muscles and encourages improved movement patterns, allowing seniors to maintain or improve their range of motion without being restrictive.

3. Support and Posture Correction

Postural Improvement: By providing subtle signals to promote better alignment and lessening pressure on muscles and joints, kinesiology tape application techniques can help correct bad posture that is frequently observed in seniors.

Improving Balance: The proprioceptive effects of the tape can help seniors become more balanced and stable, which may lower their chance of falling, which is a major worry for this population.

4. Supplemental Rehab and Wellbeing Instrument

Aide for Rehabilitation: Kinesiology tape can support specific muscles or joints in seniors receiving physical therapy or rehabilitation, which can improve the efficacy of exercises and therapies.

Inclusive Choice: Kinesiology taping is especially intriguing to seniors who prefer natural approaches to managing their health and fitness because it is a non-invasive and drug-free procedure.

5. Health of the Mind

Increased Confidence: Kinesiology tape can help seniors feel more confident about their capacity to participate in everyday activities by offering support and pain relief. This can promote independence and a positive view of their skills.

CHAPTER TWO

BASICS OF KINESIOLOGY TAPING FOR SENIORS

Fundamentals of Kinesiology Tape

Kinesiology tape's composition, elasticity, application methods, and effects on the body are all part of its principles. It's crucial to comprehend these fundamentals for seniors, in particular, to utilize technology safely and effectively.

1. Material and Composition

Stiffness: Kinesiology tape is similar to human skin in that it is made of cotton and has an acrylic adhesive that allows it to stretch longitudinally. Because of its suppleness, the tape can follow the natural contours of the body without causing discomfort.

Features That Adhere: Kinesiology tape's adhesive is made to gently stick to skin without irritating it or leaving behind residue when removed.

2. Tension and Elastic Properties

Longitudinal Stretch: Kinesiology tape allows for directed and controlled tension because it extends along its length rather than its width. This characteristic is essential for providing the appropriate amount of support without restricting mobility.

Different Stress Levels: Different application methods enable different tension levels. Whether the goal is muscle stimulation, pain alleviation, or support, tension can be changed accordingly.

3. Methods of Application

Orientation: The tape's effect on the body varies depending on which way it is applied. Depending on the intended result, tapes can be applied with stretch, without stretch, or at different tensions.

Cut and Shape: Kinesiology tape can be sliced using "cutting techniques," which allow it to be shaped into precise patterns or shapes. These patterns have several functions, including joint support, pain alleviation, and muscle facilitation.

4. The Body's Impact

Relief from Pain: Kinesiology tape, when used properly, can raise the skin, possibly relieving pressure on pain receptors and providing respite from discomfort related to a range of ailments.

Muscle Assistance and Coordination: By gently stimulating the skin's receptors, the tension of the tape can help strengthen weak muscles or make it easier for muscles to activate.

5. Precautions and Safety

Skin Precautions: In order to avoid skin problems, especially in older adults with sensitive skin, proper skin preparation, monitoring for any allergic reactions or irritation, and gentle removal techniques are essential.

Guidelines for Applications: Kinesiology tape can be used safely and effectively if users are aware of the suggested use time, tension levels, and when to seek professional advice.

6. Combining Therapy with Other Approaches

Additional Therapies: Kinesiology taping can help with movement patterns or offer further assistance with other therapies like physiotherapy or exercise regimens.

Flexibility: Its versatility makes it a flexible alternative in holistic care approaches, enabling it to be used in conjunction with other therapy modalities without interfering.

Application Techniques for Seniors

Of course! Seniors have specific needs; therefore, it's important to take those into account while using kinesiology tape.

1. Light Handling

Decreased Tension: Seniors may have more sensitive skin or a lower threshold for pressure. Use light pressure when applying the tape to offer support without hurting or irritating the skin.

Selective Positioning: Pay attention to the regions where the tape is placed. To avoid unneeded friction or discomfort, stay away from regions where skin folds appear, bony prominences, or delicate skin are present.

2. Combined Stability and Support

Securing Joints: Joint stability is a common problem for seniors. Place the tape in a way that offers support without unduly restricting joint motion. "Y-strips" and "fan cuts" are two methods that can provide support around a joint without limiting movement.

Targeted Support: Apply tape techniques that provide support without obstructing normal movement, with a focus on areas like the knees, shoulders, or lower back that are prone to discomfort or instability.

3. Techniques for Pain Management

Application Specific: When applying tape to a senior who is in pain in a specific place, use gentle lifting techniques to lift the skin and release pressure on the pain receptors.

Reduction of Pain Patterns: Apply "I-strips" or "X-patterns" to disperse stress and ease suffering, being careful that the tape doesn't tighten the skin too much or impair blood flow.

4. Adjusting Your Posture

Shoulders and Upper Back: Seniors frequently have problems with their posture. Tape should be applied in a way that gently pushes the shoulders back or promotes an upright posture to help ease the pressure on the muscles of the upper back.

Discreet Reminder: Make use of strategies like "support slings" or "posture tapes" to gently remind seniors to keep their posture correct without making them uncomfortable.

5. Enhancement of Mobility

Muscle Activation: For seniors who want to increase their mobility or participate in particular exercises, use tapping techniques that support weak muscles or help them activate their muscles.

Lower Limb Support: Methods like "calf support" or "knee stability strips" can help to stabilize and support the lower limbs when walking or engaging in other activities that require movement of the lower limbs.

6. Observation and Discussion

Practitioner Guidance: When dealing with particular mobility difficulties or chronic conditions, get help from a physiotherapist or other healthcare practitioner skilled in kinesiology taping for elders.

Regular Evaluation: Keep an eye on the elders' comfort levels and the taped areas at all times. As necessary, modify the application methods or tension to maintain healthy, irritant-free skin.

Choosing the Right Tape for Senior Skin Sensitivity

For seniors with sensitive skin, selecting the best kinesiology tape requires taking into account the tape's adhesives, materials, and hypoallergenic qualities.

1. Make-Up of Materials

Tapes Made of Cotton: Choose kinesiology tapes that are mainly composed of cotton. Compared to synthetic materials, cotton-based tapes are more pleasant, breathable, and less likely to cause irritation.

Tapes Without Latex: Because many seniors may be sensitive to latex, be sure the tape you use is devoid of latex to avoid allergic reactions.

2. Properties of Adhesion

Adhesives that are Hypoallergenic: Seek out tapes made especially for delicate skin that use hypoallergenic adhesives. These adhesives are less likely to irritate skin or trigger allergic reactions, making them friendlier.

Adhesives Based on Water: Water-based adhesive tapes are less harsh and easier on delicate skin, making them potentially more skin-friendly.

3. Comfort and Texture

Compact and pliable: Select tapes that are flexible and have a gentle texture. This guarantees comfort and lessens the possibility of abrasion or friction against the skin, which may irritate it.

Breathable Tapes: Choose tapes that let air circulate around the skin. This lessens the chance of skin irritation and helps minimize moisture buildup, especially when wearing for extended periods of time.

4. Trial & Test

Fixing Issues: Do a patch test on a small portion of the senior's skin prior to prolonged use to look for any sensitivities or negative reactions to the tape.

Test Various Brands: Not every tape that is labeled as safe for sensitive skin will necessarily be effective for every person. Try a variety of brands or varieties to see which one best suits the senior's skin type.

5. Evaluations and Suggestions

Consistent with Professional Advice: Consult therapists or medical professionals who have dealt with elderly patients and skin issues that are delicate. Based on their knowledge, they might recommend particular brands or kinds.

Reviews by Users: Seek out endorsements or reviews from people who have comparable skin sensitivity. Their firsthand knowledge can be quite helpful in determining which tapes are suitable for those with sensitive skin.

6. Methods of Application and Removal

Gentle Application: Avoid overstretching and apply the tape with the least amount of strain, especially on delicate skin or sensitive areas.

Careful Removal: To reduce skin irritation, carefully remove the tape by peeling it off in the direction that hair grows.

CHAPTER THREE

TAPING TECHNIQUES FOR COMMON SENIOR ISSUES

Taping for Joint Support and Stability

Seniors can benefit from kinesiology tape by employing particular strategies to help maintain stability and lessen discomfort while using tape for joint support and stabilization.

1. Stability of the Knee

- Utilize "X-patterns" or "Y-strips" around the knee as supportive techniques to offer stability without restricting movement. These methods can provide support for knees that are weak or rheumatic.

- **Patellar Support:** To relieve pressure and suffering related to disorders like osteoarthritis, apply a "patellar support" approach by forming a strip beneath the kneecap.

2. Stability of the Shoulder

- **Rotator Cuff Support:** Apply methods like "fan cuts" or "shoulder stability slings" to gently support the rotator cuff muscles, which will improve stability without limiting arm movement.

- **Correct Posture:** To promote improved posture and relieve shoulder pain, especially in seniors who are prone to rounded shoulders, place tape across the upper back and shoulder region.

3. Stability of Ankles

- **Ankle Stabilization:** To reduce the danger of sprains or strains, use "basket weave" or "figure-8" techniques around the ankle to minimize excessive movement and give support.
- **Arch Assistance:** Seniors with flat feet or discomfort connected to the arch can benefit from applying strips in a crisscross pattern beneath their feet to support their arch.

4. Support for Lower Back

- **Core Stability:** Use tapes in "core support" patterns to gently urge better core activation, which will help with posture and lessen strain on the lower back.
- **Lumbar Support:** To provide stability and lessen pain related to disorders like spinal arthritis, apply "vertical strips" or "spinal support" techniques down the lower back.

5. Support for the Elbow and Wrist

- **Elbow Support Relief:** Use tapes in conjunction with "elbow support techniques" to provide relief and support for the tendons impacted by ailments such as lateral epicondylitis or tennis elbow.

- Wrist Stability: Support weak wrists with methods such as "wrist stability wraps" to lessen strain when engaging in activities requiring wrist movement.

6. Help for Applications

- **Decoration of the Skin:** To guarantee optimal adherence, make sure the skin is clean, dry, and free of oils or lotions before applying the tape.

- **Gentle Tension:** Use a moderate amount of tension when applying the tape to provide support without hurting or obstructing blood flow.

- **Smooth Application:** After applying the tape, smooth it out to make sure it sticks firmly to the skin and to avoid creases that could irritate it.

Taping for Pain Relief in Arthritic Condition

Of course, applying kinesiology tape to relieve pain in arthritic situations entails methods meant to lessen discomfort and support the afflicted joints.

1. Arthritis in the Knee

- **Patellar Stabilization:** Apply strips under and around the kneecap as part of a "patellar support" procedure to relieve pressure and lessen discomfort related to knee arthritis.
- **Medial and Lateral Support:** To relieve tension and offer support to the afflicted areas, wrap "I-strips" or "X-patterns" around the sides of the knee.

2. Arthritis of the Hand and Fingers**

- **Finger Support:** To ease the discomfort associated with activities, use "basket weave" or "finger support wraps" on arthritic finger joints.
- **Thumb Stabilization:** Apply strips to the base of the thumb using methods similar to "thumb wraps" in order to decrease pain and offer support in cases of thumb arthritis.

3. Arthritis of the Hips

- **Hip Assistance:** Wrap the problematic hip joint with tape in "hip stability patterns" or "Y-strips" to provide support and reduce pain.
- **Gluteal Support:** Apply methods such as "gluteal support slings" to offer mild signals for improved alignment, which may lessen arthritis-related hip pain.

4. Arthritis of the Shoulder and Elbow

- **Shoulder Relief:** Use tapes in "fan cuts" or "shoulder stability slings" to provide support and lessen strain on the arthritis-affected shoulder joint.
- **Elbow Support:** Apply methods such as "elbow stability wraps" to reduce pain related to elbow joint arthritis.

5. Arthritic Spine Techniques

- **Spinal Support:** To provide gentle support and lessen pain related to spinal arthritis, use tapes in "spinal stability patterns" along the affected area of the spine.
- **Posture Improvement:** Reduce strain on arthritic spinal regions by using techniques such as

"posture tapes" or "core support" patterns to provide cues for improved posture.

6. Help for Applications

- **Gentle Tension**: Apply the tape with the least amount of tension possible to prevent putting further strain on delicate joints impacted by arthritis.

- **Comfortable Placement**: Make sure that the senior feels comfortable throughout daily activities and that the tape placement does not unduly restrict movement.

- **Continuous Monitoring**: Evaluate the senior's comfort level on a regular basis and modify the application or procedures in response to their comments.

Taping Strategies for Improving Mobility

With kinesiology taping, seniors can increase their mobility by using procedures that support their joints and muscles, lessen pain, and improve their movement patterns.

1. Knee Flexibility

- **Stabilizing Techniques:** To help elders with activities like walking and climbing stairs, apply "X-patterns" or "Y-strips" around the knee to provide stability without restricting movement.

- **Support for Pathell:** Use "patellar support" techniques to apply tapes under and around the kneecap in order to minimize discomfort and promote improved knee mobility.

2. Lower Back and Hip Mobility

- **Hip Support:** To support and encourage greater mobility during exercises like standing or walking, apply "hip stability patterns" or "Y-strips" around the hip joint.

- **Lumbar Assistance:** Put tapes along the lower back in "spinal stability patterns" to provide gentle guidance for better posture and less strain when moving.

3. Arm and Shoulder Flexibility

- **Support for the Rotator Cuff:** Use tapes in "fan cuts" or "shoulder stability slings" to provide support to the rotator cuff muscles, which improves arm movement without sacrificing stability.

- **Support for Wrist and Elbow:** Employ methods such as "wrist stability patterns" or "elbow stability wraps" to help in elbow and wrist movements, such as lifting or gripping objects.

4. Foot and Ankle Flexibility

- **Ankle Stabilization:** To give stability around the ankle and enhance mobility for activities like walking or standing, use "figure-8" or "basket weave" techniques.

- **Arch Support:** For seniors who experience discomfort connected to their arches, use methods like "arch support wraps" to offer mild support and promote improved foot movement.

5. Increasing Flexibility

- **Muscle Activation:** To promote better movement patterns and increased flexibility, use taping techniques that promote muscle activation, such as "muscle facilitation wraps."

- **Stretching Support:** Use tapes to help with mild stretching exercises. This will stabilize your muscles and encourage more flexibility while lowering your risk of strain.

6. Things to Consider When Applying

- **Comfortable Placement:** Make sure the tape is positioned such that seniors may move freely throughout everyday activities and that their complete range of motion is allowed without experiencing any discomfort.

- **Gradual Adaptation:** Apply taping gradually to help seniors get used to the feeling and make sure it doesn't hurt or limit their mobility.

CHAPTER FOUR

TAPING FOR SPECIFIC SENIOR BODY AREAS

Shoulders and Upper Back Taping

Of course! Seniors can address posture, shoulder stability, and discomfort issues by using kinesiology tape on their upper back and shoulders. Here are some particular methods:

1. Correcting Posture

Upper Back Support: To promote a more upright posture and lessen the strain and discomfort associated with rounded shoulders, place "Y-strips" or "posture tapes" along the upper back.

Shoulder Retraction: To enhance alignment and help elders maintain a more comfortable and natural posture, use tapes in a way that gradually draws the shoulders back.

2. Stability of the Shoulder

Rotator Cuff Support: To help with stability without restricting shoulder movement, apply "shoulder stability slings" or "fan cuts" to support the rotator cuff muscles.

Deltoid Assistance: Use methods such as "deltoid wraps" to apply tape across the deltoid muscle to help stabilize the shoulder during different exercises.

3. Pain Relieving Methods

Relief for Upper Back Pain: Put "vertical strips" or "spinal support" tapes around the upper back to ease the pain brought on by disorders such as spinal arthritis or tense muscles.

Relief of Shoulder Pain: To ease pain from arthritis or strain, apply "X-patterns" or "shoulder stability wraps" around the shoulder joint.

4. Help for Application

Gentle Tension: Use a moderate amount of tension when applying the tape to provide support without creating pain and to enable the shoulder and upper back region to move naturally.

Decoration of the Skin: To guarantee optimal adherence and comfort, make sure the skin is clean, dry, and free of lotions before applying the tape.

5. Assisting with Mobility

Improved Range of Motion: Using tapes will promote greater shoulder mobility by gently supporting muscles without limiting their range of motion when engaging in activities.

Latissimus and Pectoral Support: Apply methods like "latissimus dorsi support" or "pectoral support wraps" to help enhance the suppleness and range of motion of these muscles.

6. Expert Consultation

Medical Advice: For customized counseling, consult a physiotherapist or other healthcare practitioner with experience in kinesiology taping for certain upper back or shoulder problems.

Elbow and Forearm Taping

Of course! Kinesiology tape applied to the elbow and forearm can help elders with ailments including tennis elbow, golfer's elbow, or just general pain. Here are some particular methods:

1. Lateral epicondylitis, or tennis elbow

Treatment for Pain Relief: Apply tapes using "elbow support wraps" to relieve pain in the elbow's outer region. Relief can be obtained by "X-patterns" and "I-strips" techniques.

Muscle Activation: Apply tapes to help activate your muscles, concentrating on your forearm's extensor muscles with methods such as "muscle facilitation wraps."

2. Medial epicondylitis, or golfer's elbow)

Support Methodologies: To relieve strain and discomfort, use "elbow stability wraps" or "Y-strips" to apply tapes in a way that supports the inside section of the elbow.

Muscle Relief: To lessen golfers' elbow discomfort, apply methods like "flexor muscle support" wraps to gently support the forearm muscles.

3. Support for the Forearm

Forearm Flexor and Extensor Support: Apply tapes in "cross-patterns" or "forearm stability patterns" to provide support for the forearm's flexor and extensor muscles.

Wrist Support: During tasks requiring forearm movement, apply tapes utilizing "wrist stability techniques" to help lessen strain and discomfort in the wrist joint.

4. Help for Applications

Comfortable Placement: Make sure the tape is positioned so that mobility is possible without experiencing any discomfort, particularly when engaging in activities that require elbow and forearm motion.

Gentle Tension: To offer support without obstructing blood flow or producing discomfort, apply the tape with the least amount of tension possible.

5. Support for Movement

Improved Range of Motion: Use tapes to help elders with activities like lifting or holding objects by facilitating better elbow and forearm movement patterns.

Pain Reduction Patterns: Employ methods that attempt to gently raise the skin in order to lessen pressure on pain receptors, which will help to relieve pain and increase mobility.

6. Expert Consultation

Medical Advice: For individualized guidance about particular elbow or forearm issues, consult a physiotherapist or other healthcare professional with experience in kinesiology taping.

Knee and Lower Leg Taping

Of course! Kinesiology tape applied to the knee and lower leg can help seniors with mobility, pain, and stability problems. Here are some particular methods:

1. Support and Stability of the Knee

Patellar Stabilization: To relieve pressure and discomfort, apply tapes using a "patellar support" approach, which involves forming a supportive framework around the kneecap.

Medial and Lateral Support: For seniors with arthritis or instability in particular, apply "I-strips" or "X-patterns" down the sides of the knee to relieve strain and offer support.

2. Support for Shin and Calf

Calf Support: Use tapes to gently support the calf muscles, helping to lessen discomfort during activities. This can be done by applying them using "basket weave" or "calf support wraps" techniques.

Shin Splint Relief: Apply methods such as "shin splint wraps" to ease the pain and support the shin muscles in order to relieve shin splints.

3. Stability of Ankles

Ankle Stabilization: To provide elders with stability and support during tasks requiring ankle movement, apply tapes around the ankle in "figure-8" or "basket weave" approaches.

Achilles Tendon Support: Apply methods like "Achilles support wraps" to ease the pain and provide subtle signals for improved alignment in the Achilles tendon.

4. Methods of Pain Relief

Relief from Knee Pain: To help relieve pain, apply tape using methods that lessen pressure on pain receptors, such as "vertical strips" or "X-patterns" around the knee joint.

Lower Leg Pain: Apply tapes to the lower leg muscles to provide support without restricting motion, therefore lessening pain brought on by ailments like arthritis.

5. Help for Applying

Correct Alignment: Make sure the tape is positioned correctly to provide support without obstructing normal knee or lower leg movement.

Decoration of the Skin: Before using the tape, make sure the skin is completely clean and dry. This will provide optimal adherence and comfort, especially in delicate areas.

6. Improvement of Mobility

Improved Range of Motion: Use tapes to help elders with activities like walking and climbing stairs by facilitating better movement patterns in the lower leg and knee.

Muscle Activation: Make use of methods to help seniors stay mobile and stable while performing a variety of lower-body exercises.

7. Expert Consultation

Medical Advice: Consult a physiotherapist or other qualified healthcare provider with experience in kinesiology taping for recommendations tailored to your unique knee or lower leg problems.

CHAPTER FIVE

KINESIOLOGY TAPING FOR POSTURE IMPROVEMENT

Understanding Senior Postural Challenges

Seniors' postural difficulties are important to understand since they have an impact on their general health and wellbeing. Here are some important details regarding postural difficulties in seniors:

1. Imbalance and Weakness of Muscles

Decrease in Muscle Power: It might be difficult for seniors to maintain proper posture since they frequently see a reduction in muscular strength, especially in the postural and core muscles.

Inequality Among Muscle Groups: Seniors who experience weakness or imbalances in their muscles may take on compensatory postures, including slouching, to make up for their decreased stability.

2. Limited Range of Motion and Flexibility

Joint Stiffness: Aging-related changes, like reduced joint suppleness, can limit range of motion, making it difficult for elders to adopt and keep good posture.

Restricted Movement: Limited mobility can be brought on by illnesses like arthritis or previous injuries, which can make it difficult to move freely and have good posture.

3. Modifications to the Skeletal Structure

Changes in the Spine: Seniors may have altered cervical lordosis (pronounced inward curve of the neck) or enhanced thoracic kyphosis (rounded upper back), which can have an impact on posture.

Decrease in Bone Density: Osteoporosis and other conditions affecting bone density might increase the risk of vertebral fractures in seniors, which can impact posture.

4. Modifications to the Senses

Decreased Proprioception: The body's sense of its location in space, or proprioception, can be impacted by age-related declines in sensory perception, which can have an effect on postural control and stability

Balance and Vision Problems: Postural modifications might result in compensatory postures to preserve stability due to visual impairments or balance issues.

5. Environment and Lifestyle Effects

Limited Movement: Long periods of inactivity or sitting can weaken muscles and aggravate bad posture, particularly in older adults who spend a lot of time in back- or neck-stressing positions.

Climatic Considerations: Postural issues in elders can be made worse by poor ergonomics, such as unsupportive furniture or an inappropriate workstation configuration.

6. Psychological and Cognitive Factors

Self-Reliance and Falling Fear: Seniors who are afraid of falling may take precautionary stances that result in a stooped or bent position, which might impair their balance and general posture.

Disintegration of Thought: Due to cognitive impairment, conditions such as dementia might affect elders' ability to consciously maintain appropriate posture.

Taping Methods to Enhance Posture

Of course! Seniors' posture can be improved with kinesiology tape by using particular techniques that provide cues for improved alignment and support. These are some tactics:

1. Shoulders and Upper Back

Postural Correction: To encourage an upright posture and lessen rounded shoulders, gently draw the shoulders back using tape in the form of "Y-strips" or "posture tapes" across the upper back.

Shoulder Retraction: Support the rotator cuff muscles using exercises such as "shoulder stability slings" or "fan cuts" to help with shoulder alignment and better posture.

2. Support for the Abdominal and Core

Core Activation: Use tapes for "abdominal wraps" or "core support" to gently cue the body to activate the core more effectively, which will help you maintain an erect posture.

Ribcage Support: Help elders maintain an elevated chest for better posture by using methods that encourage ribcage expansion, such as "ribcage wraps."

3. Pelvic and Lower Back Support

Lumbar Stabilization: Use tapes in "spinal stability patterns" on the lower back to provide support and guidance on how to keep the spine neutral, which will help with better posture.

Pelvic Alignment: To improve lower back alignment, use tapes in "pelvic support" techniques to gently move the pelvis into a more neutral position.

4. Head and Neck Position

Cervical Support: Use tapes in "cervical spine support" methods to help keep the cervical curve in place, which will improve the alignment of the head and neck.

Chin Retraction: To help elders reduce forward head posture, use techniques such as "chin tucks" to gently urge them to retract their chins.

5. Help for Applying

Comfortable Placement: Make sure the tape is positioned so that it permits natural movement without creating discomfort, assisting seniors in pleasantly maintaining better posture.

Gentle Tension: Use the tape sparingly to give support without obstructing blood flow or making daily tasks uncomfortable.

6. Techniques for Postural Awareness

Mirror Feedback: Seniors can benefit from using mirrors to get visual feedback on their alignment and posture, which can help them self-correct.

Posture-Correcting activities: To reinforce improved postural habits, combine taping procedures with posture-focused activities, like light stretches or strengthening exercises.

Exercises and Taping Combinations for Postural Support

Of course! Incorporating taping techniques with exercises can greatly improve elders' postural support. Here is a mix of taping techniques and exercises:

1. Shoulder and Upper Back Exercises

Workout:

Retraction of the scapula: Pull the shoulder blades together to perform shoulder blade squeezes, whether seated or standing.

Taping: To maintain the position of the shoulder blades and promote improved posture, apply "posture tapes" or "Y-strips" across the upper back.

2. Taping the abdomen and strengthening the core

Workout:

Plank Variations: To build stronger core muscles, perform modified planks or wall planks.

Taping: Provide cues for working the core muscles while keeping an upright posture by using "core support" or "abdominal wraps".

3. Exercises for Lower Back Stability

Workout:

Posture: To build stronger gluteal and lower back muscles, do bridge exercises.

Tapping: To provide mild support and ensure correct alignment throughout the workout, apply "spinal stability patterns" throughout the lower back.

4. Training for Head and Neck Posture

Workout:

Tucks in the chin: Engage in chin tucks while seated or standing to enhance head alignment and fortify the neck muscles.

Tapping: To enhance the workout, use "cervical spine support" approaches that provide cues for keeping the cervical spine neutral.

5. Combinations of Postural Stretching and Taping Workout:

Stretch Your Chest: To counterbalance rounded shoulders and open the chest, do stretches.

Tapping: To help seniors maintain better posture, use "shoulder stability slings" or "posture tapes" to support the stretch position.

6. Incorporation into Everyday Tasks

Activity Modification: Recommend to elders that they should always sit, stand, or walk with good posture.

Tapping Support: During these exercises, use taping techniques such as "posture tapes" or "core support" to offer external support and cues for improved alignment.

7. Expert Advice and Modifications

Healthcare Consultation: To modify workouts and taping techniques to fit specific needs and limits, consult physiotherapists or other medical specialists.

CHAPTER SIX

RECOVERY AND REHABILITATION TECHNIQUES

Taping for Recovery After Exercise or Injury

Of course! Kinesiology tape can be a useful aid in seniors' recuperation following physical activity or injury. Here are several ways that tapping methods can help with the healing process:

1. Recovering Muscles

- **Reducing Fatigue:** By gently supporting and encouraging circulation, use kinesiology tape utilizing methods such as "muscle facilitation wraps" to assist in the healing of muscles.

- **Relieving pain:** Apply tape techniques like "X-patterns" or "vertical strips" to alleviate post-exercise muscle pain, facilitating a quicker recovery.

2. Support for Ligaments and Joints

- **Stabilizing Injured Joints:** Use taping techniques like "Y-strips" or "joint stability wraps" to provide support to injured or weak joints, aiding in the rehabilitation process.

- **Improving Range of Motion:** Use tapes to support the damaged area without limiting movement, enabling a regulated range of motion while performing rehabilitation exercises.

3. Handling Edema and Swelling

Support for Lymphatic Drainage: By encouraging lymphatic drainage, use taping techniques like "fan cuts" or "edema reduction techniques" to help manage swelling following an accident.

Reducing Inflammation: Gently raise the skin while applying tapes to inflammatory regions to relieve pressure, which helps to lessen inflammation and promote healing.

4. Analgesia

- **Relieving Pain** Apply taping methods, including "pain reduction patterns" or "I-strips," to provide support and subtly ease pain brought on by activity or injury.
- **Relief of Trigger Points:** Put tapes directly on sore spots or trigger points to provide targeted pain relief that will help with the healing process.

5. Considering the Application

- **Gentle Application:** To offer support without adding to discomfort or obstructing blood flow, apply the tape with the least amount of stress possible.

- **Decoration of the Skin:** Before using the tape, make sure the skin is clean and dry to promote adhesion and minimize irritation, particularly in parts of the skin that are sensitive or wounded.

6. Exercises for Progressive Recuperation

Guided Exercises: To assist in a gradual recovery and strengthening, combine taping techniques with controlled and guided exercises as suggested by a physiotherapist.

Gradual Adaptation: Modify tape techniques as healing advances, progressively diminishing support to encourage normal function of muscles and joints.

7. Expert Guidance and Observation

Medical Advice: Consult physiotherapists or medical experts for guidance on the best taping methods and workouts for your particular injury or recuperation requirements.

Enhancing Rehabilitation with Kinesiology Tape

Kinesiology tape can help seniors recover more quickly by supporting improved movement patterns, helping to activate muscles, and offering support. This is how it can improve rehabilitation:

1. Strengthening and Activating Muscles

- **Targeted Muscle Activation**: To motivate weaker muscles to contract during rehabilitation activities, use kinesiology tape in methods such as "muscle facilitation wraps".

- **Strengthening**: Use cassettes to help seniors restore their strength after surgery or injury by helping them contract their muscles during certain exercises.

2. Postural and Joint Support

- **Joint Stabilization:** To support weaker or recovering joints and facilitate rehabilitation exercises, apply taping techniques such as "joint stability wraps".

- **Postural Assistance:** Use tapes to assist good posture throughout rehabilitation exercises, making sure seniors stay in the right alignment when working out.

3. Pain Reduction and Management

- **Pain Reduction Methods:** When doing rehabilitation exercises or motions, use kinesiology tape in techniques like "pain reduction patterns" or "I-strips" to reduce discomfort.
- **Trigger Point Relief:** Tape sensitive regions to provide targeted relief; this can help minimize pain and discomfort while undergoing rehabilitation.

4. Managing Swelling and Edema

- **Edema Reduction:** Apply strategies like "lymphatic drainage methods" or "edema reduction wraps" to help control swelling or edema following rehabilitation.
- **Inflammation Reduction:** Gently raise the skin with tapes to relieve pressure on inflammatory regions and hasten the healing process.

5. Enhancing Proprioception and Range of Motion

- **Improving Proprioception:** During rehabilitation activities, seniors can benefit from tactile feedback from kinesiology tape, which can help them restore proprioception and improve their balance and coordination.
- **Facilitating Movement:** Use tapes to support movement without restricting range of motion. This

will help elders progressively restore mobility after surgery or an injury.

6. Adaptation and Gradual Progression

- **Progressive Rehabilitation:** Modify tape techniques as healing goes on, progressively diminishing support to promote normal function in the muscles and joints.

- **Customization and Monitoring:** Consult medical professionals for advice on how best to adapt taping techniques to an individual's needs and progress during their recovery.

7. Integrating Counseling Sessions with

- **Therapist Collaboration:** Arrange for the integration of kinesiology tape techniques into therapy sessions in coordination with physiotherapists or rehabilitation specialists to augment the recovery process in its entirety.

- Kinesiology tape can help with muscular activation, offer targeted support, and facilitate a more seamless healing process for elders undergoing rehabilitation programs. This can be done by caregivers and healthcare professionals.

Integration of Taping in Physical Therapy for Seniors

Senior physical therapy can benefit from the addition of taping techniques in a number of ways, including improved mobility, pain relief, and rehabilitation.

1. Evaluation and Personalization

- **Individual Assessment:** To customize taping procedures for their rehabilitation program, physiotherapists evaluate the mobility, conditions, and unique demands of elders.

- **Personalized Taping Plans:** Create customized taping plans according to the senior's injuries, limits on their range of motion, or places that need assistance during therapy.

2. Pain Reduction and Management

- **Reduction of Pain:** Include well-known pain-relieving kinesiology tape techniques to help elders feel better both during and after physical therapy sessions.

- **Localized Relief:** To provide elders with targeted pain relief during therapy, place tapes over trigger points or sensitive areas.

3. Stability and Support

- **Joint Support:** To improve stability during therapeutic exercises and motions, use taping techniques to support weak or injured joints.
- **Muscle Activation:** Use cassettes to help seniors engage particular muscle areas during focused exercises. This will help with muscle activation.

4. Enhancement of Rehabilitation

- **Improving Exercise Efficacy:** Include taping techniques to improve the efficiency of rehabilitation activities, helping elders reach improved results.
- **Improving Mobility:** Apply kinesiology tape to encourage greater proprioception and movement patterns, which will increase mobility in treatment sessions.

5. Guidance and Progressive Adaptation

- **Gradual Progression:** As seniors advance in their rehabilitation, gradually modify taping techniques, lowering support to encourage natural muscle and joint function.
- **Advice and Instruction:** Inform seniors and caregivers about the advantages of taping and

show them how to keep the tape in place or modify it for continued assistance.

6. Working together with medical professionals

- **Interdisciplinary Collaboration**: Work together to guarantee a comprehensive approach to elder rehabilitation with physiotherapists, occupational therapists, and other healthcare professionals.
- **Continuous Monitoring:** Evaluate elders' progress on an ongoing basis, modifying taping methods in response to therapy responses, and evolving rehabilitation objectives.

7. Self-Care and Empowerment

- **Self-Application Training:** Equip elders with the skills necessary to manage discomfort in between therapy sessions by teaching them how to use basic tapping techniques for continuing support.
- **Promote Self-Care:** To help elders continue their taping regimen safely, teach them how to properly prepare their skin and remove tape.

CHAPTER SEVEN

ADVANCED TAPING STRATEGIES

Advanced Techniques for Chronic Pain Management

Seniors with persistent pain may benefit from advanced kinesiology tape procedures. Here are a few sophisticated methods:

1. Decompression of the fascia

Myofascial Release: By releasing tension and increasing circulation, "fan cuts" or "webbing techniques" are used to decompress fascial layers, thereby decreasing discomfort.

Decompression in Length: Long tape strips can be used to offer continuous decompression along muscle or fascial lines, which can help relieve chronic pain.

2. Modulation of Neurosensors

Lymphatic Drainage: Apply "lymphatic strips" to help reduce swelling and encourage lymphatic drainage, which can help reduce inflammation-related pain.

Gating Mechanisms: Apply tapes in a way that elicits sensory nerve activity. This produces a gating effect that prevents the brain from receiving pain signals.

3. Stabilization of Muscle and Joint

Dynamic Stabilization: Use "functional taping techniques" to stabilize joints and muscles in a dynamic manner, supporting movement without unduly limiting it.

Proprioceptive Neuromuscular Facilitation (PNF): To enhance muscle coordination and lessen discomfort brought on by muscular imbalances, apply taping techniques that imitate PNF patterns.

4. Support Structure

Corrective Techniques: Using tapes can help correct structural abnormalities that contribute to chronic pain by promoting optimal alignment and muscle activation.

Tensegrity Applications: To redistribute pressure and lessen stress on sore areas, apply taping techniques that resemble tensegrity principles.

5. Trigger point simulation or acupuncture

Acupressure Taping: By applying tapes over trigger points or acupuncture points, you can replicate acupressure and help relieve pain by stimulating the nervous system.

Cross Taping: To promote neural inhibition and lessen pain perception, use procedures that entail crossing strips over trigger points or pain sites.

6. Ongoing Evaluation and Adjustment

Individualized Approach: Evaluate the efficacy of taping procedures on a continuing basis, modifying placements or techniques in response to seniors' pain patterns and responses.

Multimodal Integration: For all-encompassing pain alleviation, combine sophisticated taping methods with other pain-reduction tactics like exercises, modalities, or cognitive-behavioral methods.

7. Education and Professional Supervision

Expert Advice: Seek advice for managing chronic pain from skilled physiotherapists or medical specialists knowledgeable in advanced kinesiology tape procedures.

Patient Education: Enable elders to manage their chronic pain as part of their self-care routine by teaching them about the advantages and appropriate application of sophisticated taping techniques.

Taping for Balance Enhancement in Seniors

Yes, proprioceptive cues and support are provided through strategies when using kinesiology tape to improve balance in seniors. The following strategies are designed to enhance balance:

1. Stimulation of Proprioception

Ankle Stability: To enhance ankle stability and balance, use "figure-8" or "basket weave" movements around the ankles to generate proprioceptive feedback.

Arch Support for the Foot: Apply tapes in "arch support wraps" to provide indications for proper foot alignment, amplifying sensory input from the feet for greater equilibrium.

2. Support for the Core and Posture

Abdominal Activation: Encourage elders to activate their core muscles to improve stability and balance during a variety of activities by using "core support" or "abdominal wraps".

Situational Cues: To help with balance, place tapes in the form of "posture tapes" or "spinal stability patterns" down the spine to serve as subtle reminders to keep an upright posture.

3. Methods of Joint Stability

Knee and Hip Support: Apply methods such as "hip stability patterns" or "Y-strips" to support and signal improved lower body alignment, which will help with balance.

Shoulder Stability: To support the shoulders and encourage improved upper body alignment and balance, apply tape in "shoulder stability slings" or "fan cuts".

4. Exercises to Improve Balance

Taping for Exercise Support: Seniors can progressively improve their balance by using tapes to give extra support during balancing exercises without compromising the challenge.

Functional Movements: Apply taping methods to improve seniors' awareness of their balance and to offer external support as they walk or stand.

5. Mobility and Gait Training

Gait Enhancement: Use cassettes to help train your gait by giving you hints for improving your foot placement and balance when you walk or engage in other activities.

Dynamic Mobility Support: Assist elders in maintaining balance during transitions or changes in posture by utilizing approaches that provide support during dynamic movements.

6. Help for Applications

Gentle Tension: When performing balance-enhancing exercises, apply the tape with the least amount of tension possible to offer support without limiting mobility or creating discomfort.

Correct Skin Preparation: To guarantee optimal adherence and comfort, make sure the skin is clean, dry, and free of lotions before applying the tape.

7. Expert Counsel and Modification

Therapist Supervision: To guarantee correct taping techniques and modify them in accordance with specific balance issues, seek advice from physiotherapists or balance specialists.

Progressive Adaptation: As elders gain better balance, gradually reduce the amount of support provided to encourage stability and natural balance.

Combinations of Taping for Multiple Issues

Of course! For seniors managing several ailments at once, combining taping approaches can be helpful. Here's how to mix and match to solve different issues:

1. All-Inclusive Upper Body Assistance

Shoulder Stability: To help support the shoulders for stability and pain alleviation, use "X-patterns" or "shoulder stability wraps".

Postural Correction: To promote improved posture and lessen strain, place "posture tapes" or "Y-strips" along the upper back.

2. Stability and Mobility of the Lower Body

Knee Support: Apply "I-strips" or "patellar stabilization techniques" to the knees to provide extra support and alleviate pain.

Ankle Stability: To help support the ankles during mobility exercises, apply "ankle stability techniques" in figure-8 patterns.

3. Enhancing Balance and Activating the Core

Core Support: Apply "core support wraps" to encourage improved activation of the core muscles for balance and stability.

Arch Support for the Foot: Use "arch support wraps" to help improve foot alignment, which improves overall balance.

4. Joint Support and Pain Reduction

Pain Management: Apply "I-strips" or "pain reduction patterns" to targeted pain sites to provide localized relief.

Joint Stabilization: Use methods such as "Y-strips" or "joint stability wraps" to give extra support to susceptible joints.

5. Combined Posture and Mobility Enhancement

Gait Support: When walking or performing mobility exercises, employ strategies that help with gait support, such as "dynamic mobility wraps".

Posture Enhancement: Use "posture tapes" or "spinal stability patterns" to promote improved spinal alignment when moving.

6. Customization and Gradual Adaptation

Progressive Support: As elders adjust and get better, gradually reduce the amount of support provided to promote normal muscle function.

Tailored Application: For optimal effect, adjust tape locations in accordance with your demands and problem areas.

7. Expert Guidance and Observation

Healthcare Collaboration: Consult physiotherapists or other medical experts who have knowledge of senior multiple-issue taping.

Continuous Assessment: As seniors respond to the combined taping procedures, keep an eye on their development and make necessary adjustments to placements or approaches.

CHAPTER EIGHT

MAINTENANCE AND CARE

Proper Removal and Reapplication Techniques

Of course! To guarantee efficacy and avoid skin irritation, kinesiology tape removal and reapplication procedures must be done correctly. This is how you do it:

Techniques for Removal:

1. Time:

Duration: After applying the tape for three to five days, remove it to avoid causing skin irritation or adhesive buildup.

2. Process of Removal:

Slow and Gentle: To reduce pain and potential skin irritation, remove the tape slowly and softly, following the direction in which hair grows.

Warmth Application: To help loosen the adhesive and make it easier to peel off, use a damp, warm cloth or take a warm shower prior to removal.

3. Removal of Adhesive:

Surfactant Debris: Use oil (such as baby oil or olive oil) to gently rub the region to remove any adhesive residue that may have remained on the skin after removal.

4. After Removal: Skin Care

Skin Inspection: After removal, look for any indications of redness or irritation on the skin. Reapply the tape after giving the skin time to air and heal.

Reapplying Strategies:

1. Skin Assessment:

Dry and Clean: To achieve the best adhesion, make sure the skin is clean, dry, and free of oils, lotions, or perspiration before reapplying the tape.

Surface Free: Shave the region for at least 12 hours before applying the tape if hair removal is necessary to avoid irritating the skin.

2. Application of Tape:

Gentle Tension: To prevent limiting blood flow or creating discomfort when moving, apply the tape with the least amount of tension possible.

Smooth Application: To guarantee correct adherence without creases or wrinkles, gently smooth the tape onto the skin.

3. Modification and Revision:

Avoid Overlapping: To avoid exerting too much pressure or causing irritation, carefully align the edges of the tape rather than overlapping them when applying it again.

Repositioning: To obtain the required amount of coverage or support without creating discomfort, realign the tape as needed while applying.

4. After-Applicant Handling

Inspection of the Skin: After reapplication, keep an eye out for any indications of redness or irritation on the skin. If irritation arises, remove the tape right away.

Allow Adhesion Time: To guarantee best adhesion, let the tape a few hours to properly adhere before engaging in strenuous activity.

Caring for Skin When Using Kinesiology Tape

When using kinesiology tape, it's important to take care of the skin to avoid irritation and preserve skin health. Here are some vital pointers:

Prior to Tape Application:

1. Skin Assessment:

Hygiene: Prior to using the tape, make sure the skin is clean and dry. After properly cleaning the area with moderate soap and water, pat it dry.

Avoid Lotions/Oils: As they may impair adhesive adhesion, avoid putting lotions, oils, or creams on the skin prior to taping.

While Applying Tape:

2. Courtesy Use:

Minimal Tension: To avoid putting too much strain on the skin and to encourage comfort and healthy circulation, apply the tape with a light tension.

Avoid Stretching: When putting the tape on, try not to strain it too much, as this may irritate and hurt your skin.

After Applying Tape:

3. Inspection of the Skin:

Surveillance Skin: Keep an eye out for any indications of redness, itching, or irritation on the skin beneath the tape. If there are any negative reactions, take off the tape right away.

Permit Skin to Exhale: Refrain from leaving the tape on for too long. Every few days, take off and reapply the tape to give the skin a chance to breathe and heal.

Treatment of Skin in Between Applications:

4. Accurate Elimination:

Gentle Peeling: To reduce skin irritation, peel off the tape slowly and gently, following the direction in which hair grows.

Warmth Application: Before removing tape, a warm shower or the application of a warm, damp cloth might help soften the adhesive and facilitate peeling off.

5. Removal of Adhesive Residue:

Gentle Cleaning: After removing the tape, carefully rub off any leftover adhesive residue using oil (such as baby oil or olive oil). Then, wash the area with a moderate amount of soap and water.

Patience in Removing Residue: Be patient, and take your time to remove any adhesive residue to prevent rubbing too hard and irritating your skin.

6. Human Humidity:

Moisturize Gently: To keep the skin hydrated, especially if it dries out easily, moisturize with a light, hypoallergenic lotion after cleansing.

Overall Things to Think About:

Correct Fit and Position: Make sure the tape is applied appropriately, avoiding any folds or creases that can irritate or hurt the skin.

Awareness of Skin Sensitivity: Keep any allergies or sensitivities to your skin in mind. Seniors who suffer from chronic discomfort might want to think about using silicone-based or hypoallergenic adhesives.

Frequency and Duration of Taping for Senior Individuals

Seniors' kinesiology taping frequency and duration might vary depending on a number of aspects, such as the tape's intended use, the patient's needs, and skin sensitivity. The following general rules apply:

Surveillance:

1. Use in Short Term:

Every Couple of Days: It may be sufficient to apply kinesiology tape every few days for acute problems or temporary support. It stops long-term adhesion and lets the skin breathe.

2. Extensive Assistance:

Many Times Every Week: Seniors may find it helpful to reapply the tape every two to three days to maintain its effectiveness and prevent skin irritation in cases of continual support or chronic problems.

Length:

1. Serious Problems:

From a few days to a week: When treating an acute problem, using kinesiology tape for a few days to a week may be enough to relieve the symptoms.

2. Static Situations or Assistance:

Personal Use: Seniors may use kinesiology tape frequently for several weeks or longer, with brief intervals to enable the skin to heal, for persistent ailments, or for continuing support.

Taking into Account:

Sensitivity to Skin: Seniors who have sensitive skin may require shorter durations or more frequent changes to avoid irritation.

Evaluation and Tracking: Check the skin frequently for any indications of irritation or negative reactions. If any skin problems occur, take off the tape and give your skin time to heal before applying it again.

Purpose of Taping: The duration and frequency of tape application can be determined by the purpose (pain alleviation, support, or improved mobility). Observe any particular guidance that a medical practitioner provides.

Overall Advice:

Application Area Rotation: To avoid causing skin irritation or possible sensitization, avoid taping the same area over and over.

Treatment of Skin in Between Applications: To preserve skin health and reduce irritation, make sure to take adequate care of your skin both before and after taping.

Professional Advice: Based on unique demands and situations, get advice from physiotherapists or other medical specialists to determine the optimal frequency and duration.

CHAPTER NINE

CASE STUDIES AND REAL-LIFE EXAMPLES

Successful Applications in Senior Individuals

Kinesiology tape has the potential to be quite beneficial for senior citizens, providing a range of advantages for a variety of ailments or issues. Here are a few examples of effective applications:

1. Relieving Pain:

Inflammation: When applied to arthritic joints, taping techniques can provide support without limiting movement and relieve discomfort and inflammation.

Strains in Muscles: The pain-relieving qualities of kinesiology tape can help seniors who have overuse injuries or muscular strains.

2. Correcting Posture:

Correct Posture: By offering cues for alignment and support, tapping techniques can help seniors maintain better posture and lessen the strain on their shoulders and back.

Balance Enhancement: Methods that encourage more stability and alignment might help people feel more balanced when going about their everyday business.

3. Improvement of Mobility:

Gait Improvement: Kinesiology tape can help elders maintain appropriate walking patterns and lessen discomfort by supporting gait training.

Joint Stability: Support and stability can be provided by applications around joints, such as the knees and ankles, which improve mobility and lower the chance of injury.

4. Assistance with Rehabilitation:

Activation of Muscles: When performing rehabilitation activities, tapping techniques can help activate weak muscles, which can help recover strength and function.

Controlling Pain During Treatment: Seniors can perform rehabilitation exercises more easily by using kinesiology tape to reduce discomfort during therapy sessions.

5. Reduction of Edema:

Drainage of the Lymph: Lymphatic flow-promoting techniques can help manage edema following surgery or injury, assisting in the reduction of swelling and the promotion of recovery.

6. Assistance During Tasks:

Daily Support: When engaging in different daily activities, such as walking, gardening, or light exercise, kinesiology tape can offer extra support.

7. Advantages for Psychology:

A feeling of safety: Kinesiology tape can give seniors the extra support they need to participate in activities with greater comfort and confidence.

8. Improved Standard of Living:

Improved Comfort: Applications that are successful can result in less discomfort, more mobility, and better posture, all of which can enhance the quality of life for seniors overall.

Taking into Account:

Personal Differences: Depending on the individual's demands, skin sensitivity, and the particular ailment being treated, kinesiology tape applications can have varying degrees of success.

Professional Guidance: Speaking with physiotherapists or other medical experts guarantees appropriate application methods catered to seniors' particular needs.

Personal Testimonials and Experiences

Since I don't keep or access individual data or real-life events, I don't have access to personal testimonies or unique experiences. But I can provide some anecdotal or broad beneficial experiences that people have had with kinesiology tape:

1. Relieving Pain:

Reduced Discomfort: Some people report feeling less pain and discomfort, particularly in places where they are more likely to get sprains or strains in their joints or develop chronic pain problems like arthritis.

2. Enhanced Performance and Mobility:

Enhanced Movement: Thanks to kinesiology tape's support during physical activities, athletes and energetic people frequently report increased flexibility and performance.

3. Support for Posture:

Better Alignment: When employing taping techniques centered on postural support, many users report better posture and less strain on the shoulders and back.

4. Healing and Recuperation:

Easier Recuperation: Kinesiology tape can help people suffering from injuries or undergoing rehabilitation by promoting muscular activation, decreasing edema, and hastening healing.

5. Advantages for Psychology:

Sense of Security: People who wear kinesiology tape report feeling more confident and secure in their movements, which they attribute to the additional support.

6. Convenience Throughout Activities:

Increased Comfort: People who are elderly or have mobility problems may have more comfort and support during everyday tasks, which enables them to be more independent.

7. Non-Disruptive Assistance:

Unrestricted Assistance: Kinesiology tape's non-invasive design, which offers support without restricting movement or producing discomfort, is something that many users find appealing.

Challenges and Solutions in Kinesiology Taping for Seniors

Seniors have distinct considerations when it comes to kinesiology taping, such as skin sensitivity, mobility limitations, and a range of health disorders. As such, there may be particular challenges. The following problems and possible fixes are listed:

Difficulties:

1. Sensitivity to Skin:

Problem: Seniors frequently have sensitive skin that is prone to allergies or irritation, which increases the risk of adhesive-related skin problems.

2. Restricted Movement:

Problem: Seniors with mobility impairments may find it difficult to apply or remove tape on their own, particularly in difficult-to-reach places.

3. Intricate Medical Conditions:

Problem: Seniors may have a variety of health problems, making the application more difficult because of things like scars, brittle skin, or different degrees of pain.

Remedies:

1. Skin Selection and Preparation:

A remedy: To lessen skin sensitivity, use silicone-based or hypoallergenic tapes. Prioritize thorough skin preparation, and before applying a full treatment, conduct patch tests to gauge skin sensitivity.

2. Helped Submission:

A remedy: Helping seniors put on or take off tape may be beneficial. Family members, caregivers, and healthcare professionals can assist in ensuring appropriate application and removal methods.

3. Customized Methods:

Solution: Customize tape methods according to each person's unique health issues and skin integrity. Apply with more care, modifying the tension and positioning to suit areas that are delicate or damaged.

4. Academic Assistance:

A remedy: Give seniors instructional materials or training on how to handle and maintain kinesiology tape properly.

Provide advice on how to take care of your skin, apply it again, and spot symptoms of skin irritation.

5. Expert Counseling

Solution: To ensure safe and efficient taping techniques, seek advice from medical specialists, phys otherapists, or occupational therapists with expertise working with elders.

6. Alternative Approaches to Assistance:

A remedy: Instead of depending only on kinesiology tape, consider additional support options, including braces, compression clothing, or other assistive equipment that provides comparable advantages.

Verdict:

Seniors with particular issues demand a customized strategy when it comes to kinesiology taping. Successful and comfortable use depends on prioritizing skin health, providing support during application, and adjusting approaches according to individual needs. Seeking expert guidance and imparting appropriate knowledge on tape usage will greatly improve seniors' kinesiology taping experience and efficacy.

CONCLUSION

Although kinesiology taping has a wide range of potential benefits, it also offers some unique obstacles when applied to the elderly population. Several key features were clear throughout the course of our investigation, illuminating the potential and limitations of using kinesiology tape for this population.

Advantages and Prospects:

Kinesiology tape is a flexible tool for addressing a wide range of geriatric health issues. It has a wide range of applications, including arthritic pain alleviation, improved posture, increased mobility, and assistance during rehabilitation. There have been reports of successful applications leading to less pain, better mobility, better posture, and psychological reassurance, all of which contribute to an increase in the quality of life for the elderly.

Impediments Encountered

However, obstacles exist, particularly regarding skin sensitivity, limited movement, and complex health concerns. Many elderly people have sensitive skin that can respond negatively to adhesive. Mobility difficulties may also make it difficult to apply or remove the tape on one's own. In addition, older adults may present with a range of health issues that call for individualized approaches that protect the unique characteristics of their skin.

Strategies such as skin preparation: The use of hypoallergenic tapes, and the provision of aided application can help patients overcome these obstacles. Safe and effective application requires individualized methods, instruction for the elderly, and expert advice. In addition to, or as a replacement for, kinesiology tape, other forms of support exploration may reveal useful alternatives.

Future Prospects:

Finally, kinesiology taping's potential to aid seniors in a variety of ways without resorting to intrusive measures cannot be overstated. Customized techniques, education, and expert advice can pave the way for more successful and comfortable usage despite obstacles such as skin sensitivity, mobility restrictions, and health complexity. Safe and effective use of kinesiology tape among the elderly requires an emphasis on skin health, assistance with application, and individualization of procedures. Improved outcomes and more pleasant experiences for seniors who seek its advantages will be the result of continued collaboration among caregivers, healthcare professionals, and seniors themselves.